INTERMITTENT FASTING

I0408144

The Fast Diet Plan to Weight Loss Success & Longevity

Stephany J. Greene

1st Edition, 2017

Table of Contents

Introduction

Intermittent fasting has been the secret of health since time immemorial. It has always been in practice throughout the history of human beings, mainly as a religious practice. However, these days it has a different meaning, one that is focused more on health and dieting. Science also widely agrees upon the fact that eating less or going on period of fasting, is likely to increase longevity in healthy human beings. All the more reason to explore the usefulness and practicalities of intermittent fasting.

Currently, many individuals are rediscovering this dietary involvement. And not just because it can bring spiritual enlightenment, but more so because of health reasons. If intermittent fasting is done the right way, it can indeed bring numerous benefits to the human body. We will explore this topic thoroughly throughout this book.

Before delving into the details, however,it's important to understand exctly what we are talking about. So what exactly is intermittent fasting? In essence, it is a balance plan of eating, where there are individual cycles between periods of fasting and eating. Intermittent fasting does not state which types of foods a person should eat, but rather the time at which you should eat them. In respect to this, it should be stated clearly that intermittent fasting is technically not a "diet," but it is more accurately described as an "eating pattern".

Many people are already fasting each and every day, while they are sleeping. Yes, that also can be referred to as fasting – after all, we call our first meal of the day breakfast for a reason, right? Breakfast literally has the meaning in the word: to break the fasting. Intermittent fasting can be as simple as prolonging that fast slightly longer. It can be achieved by not taking breakfast and eating your first meal at noon and the last meal at 8 pm in the night. Then you are practically fasting for sixteen hours every day and having an eight-hour eating window. But this is just one of the methods of fasting we willxplore in this book.

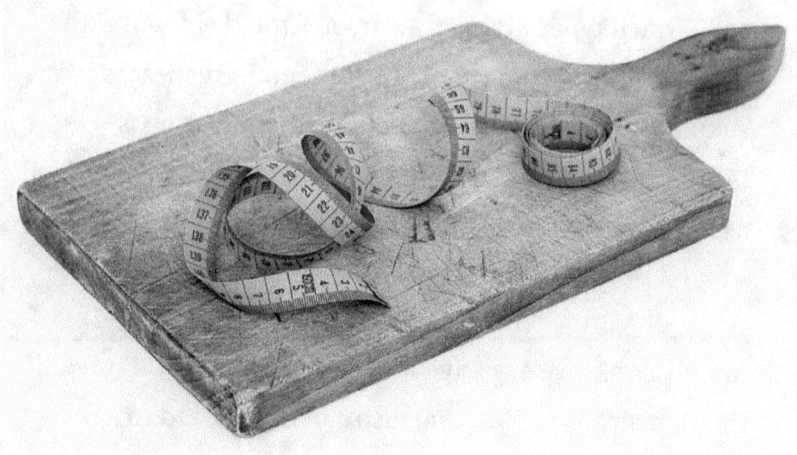

Fasting truly means eating nothing and losing weight that way

In spite of what you may think, intermittent fasting is very simple to do. That is, after the first few hours of agony where your body needs to adapt. Many individuals report having more energy while fasting and also generally feel better. Hunger is typically not that huge of an issue, even though it can be a big challenge initially, while the body is getting used to not eating for lengthened time frames. No food is permitted amid the fasting time frame; however, you can drink coffee, water, tea and other types of non-caloric refreshments. This is also a big difference from religious fasting, where this is often not permitted.

A few types of intermittent fasting permit little measures of low-calorie foods, while on the fasting period. It is allowed that an individual can take supplements while fasting, so long as calories are not present in them.

How Does Intermittent Fasting Work?

At its extreme core, fasting essentially permits the body to smolder off body fats that are in excess. It is essential to realize that this is ordinary. The human body has adapted to the requirement for energy. Fats of the body are just food energy that has been kept away. If you don't eat, your body will basically "eat" its fat for energy. This used to be quite useful back when we hunted animals and gathered foods in the wild (you know, back in the Stone Age), but in a society of abundance, this has become somewhat of a health issue for some people.

It doesn't mean anybody's genes are bad, it simply means genes have evolved in a way that's no longer applicable in a society of abundance. In fact, you could argue that if you store masses of fat, your genes are superior!

However, we must go back to the time where those genes are useful, and emulate the scarcity of food that was present for many tens of thousands of years in the past. Yes, intermittent fasting basically simulates the society of hunter-gatherers, where food was not as omnipresent as it is in today's world. This is the exact reason why it can be so damn powerful for some people.

The Inner Workings

Life is about balance. This also applies to eating and fasting. Fasting, when all things considered, is just the other side of eating. Simply put: If you are not eating, you are fasting. Let's just explore the means by which intermittent fasting works.

When we eat, more food vitality is ingested than can instantly be utilized. Some of this energy must be put away for later utilization. This means, our body stores the excess energy we take in during the day, and stores it in our bodies as fat mass.

Insulin is the primary hormone required in food energy storage, and the liver plays a primary role in this biological procedure. That looks a little bit like the following:

Eat Food ➡ Increase Insulin ➡ Store Sugar in Liver
Produce Fat in Liver

When we eat, insulin rises, thus assisting in the storage of energy that is in excess in two separate ways. Sugars can be coupled into extensive chains, which we call *glycogen*. These glycogens contain a LOT of energy. When having eaten more food than our energy requires, our body deems the excess glycogens to be 'too much'. So what does the body do? Naturally, it decides to store the glycogen in the liver. And that is where fat is produced, the storage chamber of the body's energy.

There is, nonetheless, a limited amount of storage room for sugars; and the moment that is achieved, the liver begins to transform the glucose that is in excess into fat. This procedure is well-known in science as *De-Novo Lipogenesis* (which means 'Making Fat from New').

How Fat Is Made

Some of the fat that is newly created is directly stored in the liver. However, the greater part of the fat is sent out to other fat deposits within the human body. Because this is a very complicated process, there is no restriction to the measure of fat that can be produced.

Thus, there are two corresponding food energy storage frameworks that exist in the human bodies. One of the food energy storage systems accessible with a lot of ease however it has restricted storage room (glycogen), and the other is very hard to get to yet it has boundless storage room (body fat).

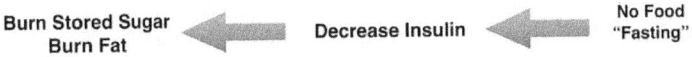

The procedure goes backward when we don't eat (fasting). The levels of insulin fall, flagging the body to begin burning the energy that is stored, since there is no more energy coming through from the food we used to eat. The body now has to haul glucose out of the storage areas, so as to burn for energy since the blood glucose has fallen.

When this sugary source of energy is depleted, that is when you can start losing body fat. You're absolutely right: the body's fat reserves are only reverted to in an extreme situation. And that's when no other energy source is available. Fasting is the tool we can use which can get us to this point of losing body fat.

Understanding Energy in Dieting

As we discovered in this chapter, the most effortlessly accessible source of energy is glycogen. However, it's a little more complicated than that. To provide energy that helps our body cells to function, glycogen is broken down into glucose molecules. This can give the body enough energy to control itself for about 24-36 hours. From that point onward, the body will begin breaking down fat for vitality. In this transition phase, the body just truly exists in two states of burning energy – the regular state of being, where the level of insulin is high, as well as the fasted state when insulin is low. Individuals are either storing food energy, or burning it.

There will be no net gain of weight if eating and fasting are balanced. In case we begin eating, the moment we come out of bed and do not seize until we go to sleep, we invest all our day in the state of being where we have plenty of energy. After some time, this means we will put on weight.

We have not given an opportunity to our body to burn food energy.

To shed pounds or to reestablish balance, we need to add the amount of time we burn food energy (fasting). Fasting permits the body to utilize its stored energy. The critical thing to comprehend, is that there is nothing wrong with that. Our bodies are designed that way. That is the thing that bears, cats, dogs, and lions do. That is what we humans do, as all mammals will.

Considering a situation where an individual is constantly eating, then the body will utilize the incoming food energy and will never burn the body fat and will continue to be stored. The body will save the body fat for the instance where there is no ingesting taking place and thus creating a lack of balance.

Breaking free from the state of being where we eat all the time is challenging. But it is not impossible. With some guidance, everybody can achieve this, but relatively good health is indeed required for this method of food indigestion. Let's explore some ways in which we can start our fasting challenge.

Methods to Intermittent Fasting

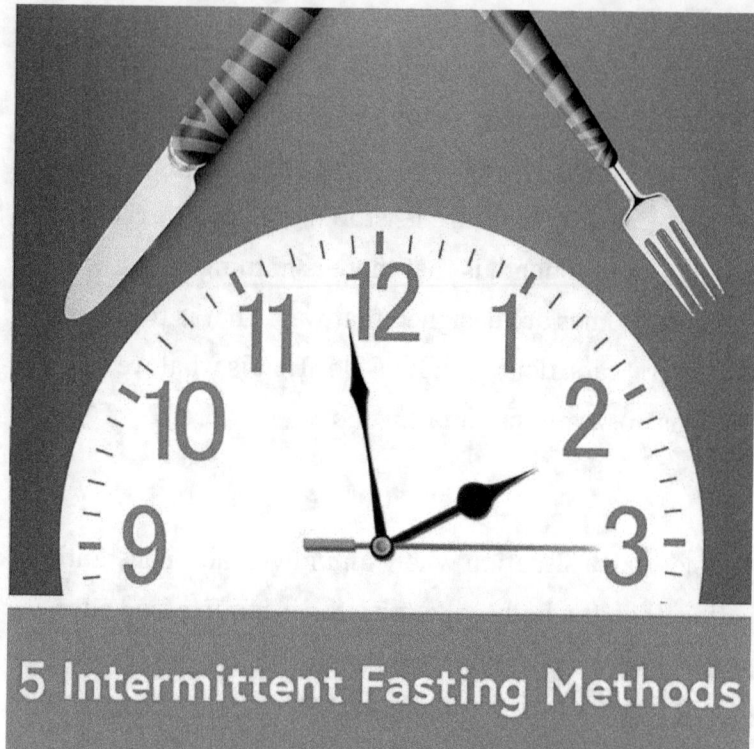

5 Intermittent Fasting Methods

There exist about five regularly used dieting methods for intermittent fasting. However, each and every technique will yield better outcomes for various individuals. Researchers clearly outline that you should not force oneself to tail a specific technique, because it is not going to go as expected. Everybody is different, and one body will respond differently to a method than another. Pick a method that makes <u>your</u> life simpler. Otherwise, the yields of your fasting might be short-term.

So, how exactly do we discover what's best for ourselves? Every technique has its particular rules for to what to eat and what extent to fast amid the "eating" stage. We will discuss the most well-known techniques and the fundamentals of how they function.

Remember, intermittent fasting is not for everybody, and those with health situations of any sort ought to check with their physician before switching up their normal schedule. It is likewise critical to identify that individual objectives and way of life are key components to consider while picking a fasting method.

The Leangains Method

Suitable for: Dedicated individuals who regularly go to the gym, who desire to both gain muscle and burn body fat efficiently.

How this method works: Fast for fourteen hours (ladies) to sixteen hours (men) each and every day for a set period of time (for example, two weeks at a time). After the fasting period, "eat" for the other eight to 10 hours. Amid the fasting time frame, an individual should devour no calories; however, you can have sugar-free gum, calorie-free sweeteners, black coffee, and diet soda. A little milk in your black coffee will not do harm, either.

Many people will think that it's least demanding to fast during night time and into the morning hours, ending the fast around six hours after breaking from sleep. This timetable is versatile to whichever individual's way of life, yet keeping up a steady eating window period is essential. Something else to consider is this: hormones in the body can get off balance and thus make it more difficult adhering to the program. Especially females with hormonal imbalances could be impacted by this matter.

When and what you eat whilst in the eating period likewise relies on upon the exercising duration of an individual. During your workout days, carbs are more important to eat than fat. On days that you rest, the intake of fat ought to be higher. Consumption of protein ought to be genuinely high consistently each day; however, it will differ depending on the objectives, gender, age, body fat mass and exercising levels. Notwithstanding your particular program, natural foods ought to make up the greater part of your calorie consumption. However, when there is no the opportunity for a dinner, protein shakes, or feast substitution bar is allowed.

Pro's: For some, the best part of this program is that on the majority of the days, meal recurrence is unimportant — an individual can truly eat at whatever point you feel like it, but this must be inside the eight-hour "eating" phase. All things considered, a great number of people find it easier breaking the eating period of the fasting into three separate meals and stick to it; since we are ordinarily as of now customized to eat along these lines.

Cons: However, there is adaptability in when you eat; Leangains normally has a particular set of rules for what types of foods to eat, particularly in connection to when you are exercising. The exacting nutrition strategy and meal planning around exercising sessions can make the program somewhat harder to stick to. However, the results will be visible faster and you will certainly feel a lot healthier in a short time span. Also make sure you are in a relatively healthy condition with your body before starting this intensive training method, otherwise you might wear yourself out.

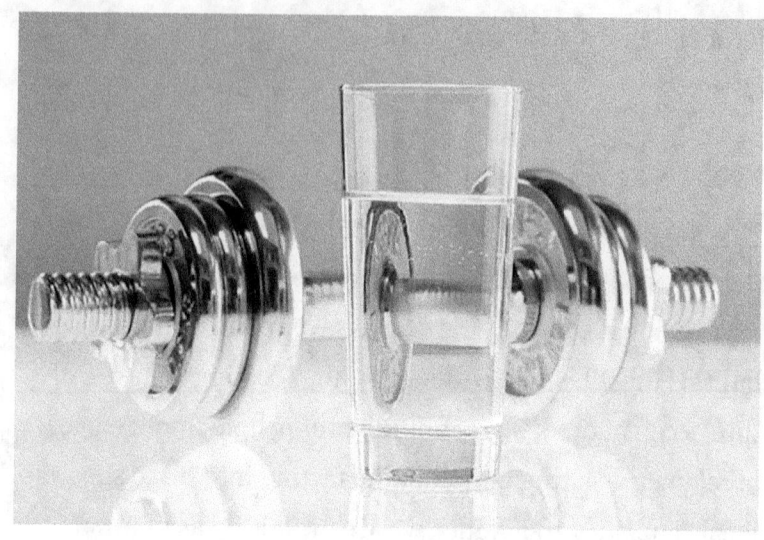

Drink water and hit the gym whilst fasting

Eat, Stop, Eat

Suitable for: People who can tolerate changing diets, mainly desiring to lose body fat.

How this method works: Go without eating for 24 hours on one or more occasion for every week. No food at all is ingested; however, one can drink refreshments that are free from any calories. Immediately when the fast has ended, you then return to eating regularly. Some people require completing the fast at an ordinary eating time with a major meal, while other persons are fine finishing the fast with evening goodies.

The primary rational? Consuming food along these lines will diminish the general consumption of calories without truly constraining what one is capable of eating — exactly how regularly, as per *Eat Stop Eat*-technique. It is essential to know that consolidating frequent exercises, especially resistance exercises, is vital to prevailing on this strategy if the reduction of weight or enhanced body organization are the main objectives.

Pro's: While to many individuals, twenty-four hours may appear like quite a while to stay without eating, the flexibility of this program is the greatest news. You do not need to go full blast at the start. Go as long as of you are capable of without eating the first day and step by step increment fasting times to become longer. This is perfect to help the body adjust. It is highly recommended to start the fast on a day where you have no eating commitments (like for a date or party time) and when you are occupied.

This technique has no "prohibited foods," and no counting calories, measuring foodstuffs or confining your diet, which somewhat makes it less demanding to adhere to it. Regardless, you need to eat like an average adult. It is simply about balance: You can, however, eat whatever you desire, but not too much of it (A piece of pie is okay, however, the entire pie is not).

Cons: Going a longer period of time with no calories might be excessively hard for some — particularly at first. A huge number of individuals battle with having extended time frames without food, bringing up irritation signs and other symptoms, including headaches, weariness, or having a grumpy feeling or restless (however, the side effects can clear off after some time).

The long periods of fasting can likewise make it tempting to fling after a fast. It can be effectively settled. It takes a considerable measure of self-control, a virtue which some people do not have.

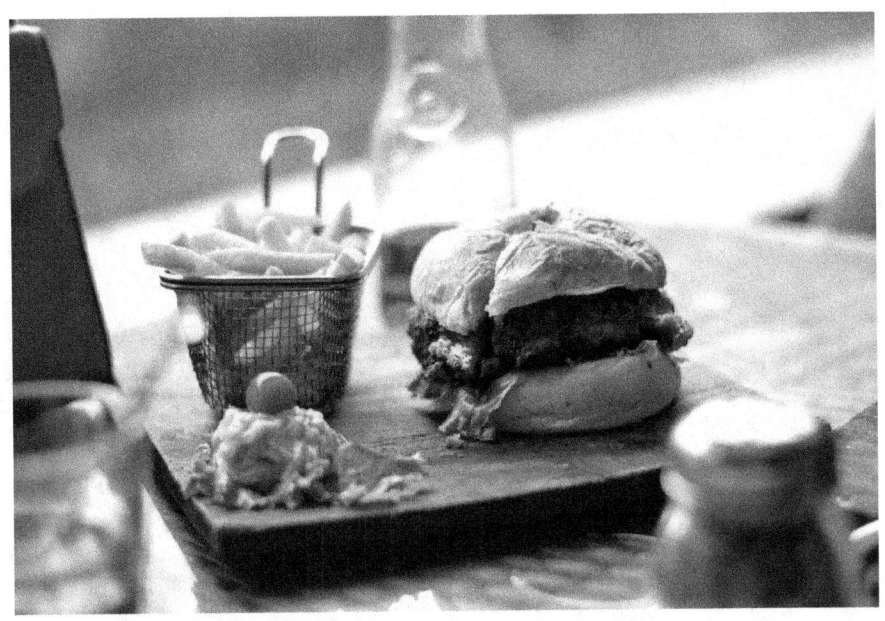

An example of a tempting meal, avoid this after the fast

The Warrior Diet

<u>**Suitable for:**</u> Persons who like adhering to rules whist dieting.

<u>**How this method works:**</u> Warriors-in-training might hope to go without eating for around twenty hours consistently each day and eat a big meal each evening. Whatever you would like, eat it, and that huge feast is likewise essential to the strategy. The rationality there depends on eating the supplements the body requires in a

state of harmony with day-to-day rhythms. It also goes by the fact that humans are nighttime eaters, characteristically customized for night eating.

The duration of fasting for this diet is truly about "under eating". An individual can eat a couple of portions of crude organic product or veggies, freshly pressed fruit juice, and a couple of servings of protein, if craved during the 20-hour fast. The eating phase (that lasts for four hours) is during the night, so as to expand the ability of the *Parasympathetic Nervous System*. This assists the body recover, it promotes inner calmness, digestion, and relaxation, whilst likewise permitting the body to utilize the supplements ingested for body repairs and development.

Consuming food during night time may also assist the body to deliver hormones and burn fat in the day time. It is highly recommended to begin with, veggies, fat, and protein. After completing those food groups, just on the off-chance that you are still hungry, you can eat foods with a bit more starch or fat in them.

Pro's: Many individuals have inclined toward this eating regimen since the period of "fasting" still permits the fasting person to consume a couple of little snacks, which might make it much simpler to complete the fast. As this approach clarifies (and the "examples of success stories" part of *The Warrior Diet* site underpins), numerous physicians likewise report exponential increment of energy levels and loss of fat.

Cons: The rules for what an individual should eat (and when) has proven to be difficult to follow long-term, although it is pleasant to eat a couple of snacks as opposed to abandon any food calories for 20 or more hours. It will make it more tempting to get off track and simply start eating again.

The tight schedule and food plan may likewise meddle with get-togethers, which might be tricky for a few. Moreover, ingestion of a single main meal during the night — while adhering to the rules of what to feed on, and in whatever manner of arrangement — can be hard, particularly for the individuals who favor not to consume large meals late at night, or find that hard to stomach.

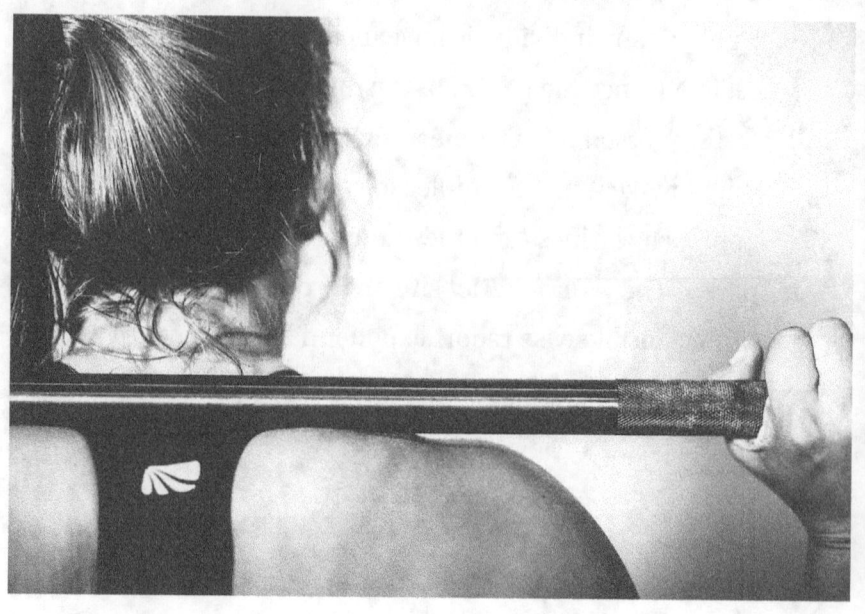

Fitness motivates the mind to start losing weight

Fat Loss Forever

Suitable for: Gym rats who cherish cheat days in diets.

How this method works: Not totally happy with the diets of intermittent fasting as mentioned previously? The *Fat Loss Forever* technique takes the most effective parts of methods like *Leangains*, *Eat Stop Eat*, and *The Warrior Diet*, and consolidates everything into a single awesome plan. An individual likewise gets a single cheat day every week (yippee!) — trailed by a fast of 36 hours (boo!). From that point forward, the rest of the seven-day cycle is divided between the distinctive fasting conventions.

It is highly recommended to save the longest fasts for the days that you are most busy, permitting you to concentrate on gaining and abstain from concentrating on hunger. The arrangement likewise incorporates exercising programs (utilizing bodyweight and free weights) to assist members to achieve most extreme fat losses in the least complex way that could be available. Yes, this method is mostly for those hardcore people that want change fast. But it is also the method that will get you results the quickest, by far.

Pros: In accordance with various researchers, despite the fact that everybody is fasting each day — amid the time when we are not feeding — the vast majority of us do as such erratically, which makes the receiving of the benefits more difficult. This technique gives a weekly plan for fasting for the body get used to this organized schedule and receive the full advantage from the time frames for fasting.

Cons: On the other side, if one experiences serious difficulty cheat days in a healthy way (i.e. having the capacity to enjoy balance and switch off that green light when now is the ideal time), this strategy may not be for you. It might also be difficult to take the 36-fasting punishment after the cheat day for some people.

Moreover, because the arrangement is entirely particular and the fasting/eating plan differs each and every day, this strategy can be somewhat confounding to take after. In any case, the arrangement comes with a calendar, taking note of how an individual should fast and practice every day, which might ensure the technique is simpler.

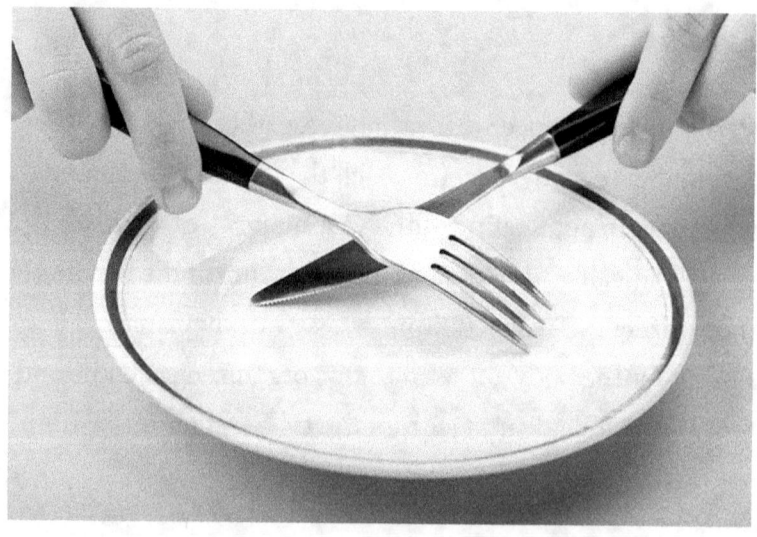

Fasting means an empty plate on certain moments

UpDay / DownDay Diet

Also known as: *Alternate-Day Diet*, or *Alternate-Day Fasting*

Suitable for: Dieters who are disciplined with a particular objective.

How this method works: It is simple: Feed on almost nothing or very small amounts on a single day, and eat like ordinary on the next day. During the low-calorie days, that implies one fifth of your ordinary calorie ingestion. So utilizing 2,000 or 2,500 calories (for ladies and men, in that order) as a guide that implies a "fasting" (or "down") day ought to be 450 to 50 calories. Individuals can utilize this technique to make sense of what number of calories to ingest on the day of low-calorie consumption.

To ensure that "down" days are simpler to adhere to, it is highly recommended to opt for food supplanting shakes, since they're braced with fundamental supplements and can be consumed for the duration of the day instead of split into little meals.

For this, I recommend you to look into information about protein shakes and different types of (crushed food) smoothies. However, that goes beyond the scope of this book and is a complete topic in its own. In any case, meal substitution shakes ought to just be utilized during the initial two weeks of the eating regiment — from that point forward, you ought to begin eating genuine foodstuffs on "down" days. The following day, eat like ordinary.

Note: In a situation where exercising is part and parcel of an individual's routine, one might find it difficult to go for training sessions on the days of lower calorie consumption. It might be brilliant to keep any exercises on those days on the friendlier side, or spare workout sessions for your ordinary calorie days.

Pro's: This technique is about the reduction of weight; therefore, if that is your primary objective, this is one to look into closely. Averagely, the individuals who burn calories by 20% to 35% witness a loss of around 2 pounds for every seven days.

Cons: Whereas the technique is quite simple to do, it might be anything but difficult to overdo on the "ordinary" day. An ideal approach to remain on the right path is preparing the meals ahead of time as frequently as would be prudent. Therefore you are not gotten at the drive-through or whatever you-can-eat buffet with a protesting stomach.

Food for Thought

While these five strategies are the most popular regarding incorporating sessions of fasting into your eating plan, there are numerous other comparative methods of insight given meal timing. For the individuals who incline toward a less inflexible strategy, there is additionally the idea of ingesting foodstuffs instinctively. Nevertheless, some trust this has the capability of prompting gorging or over ingestion of calories.

Obviously, fasting — whichever the technique used — is not for everybody. On the off chance that you have any restorative conditions, special dietary prerequisites, or serious diseases, it's helpful and even highly recommended to seek advice from a specialist before fasting.

It requires our body some period of time to change to the necessary conditions, and some require more time than others. Always remember that hormones can make it harder for ladies to adhere to fasting arrangement than for men. Females should always begin gradually and with a shorter fast than men for these hormonal reasons. Finally, in case intermittent fasting does not make you feel better than before, take a stab at something else, or acknowledge the way that is possibly fasting is not for you.

5 Tips for Starting the First Fast

In case you do try out fasting, remember these general tips:

1. **Drink a lot of water**. Remaining well hydrated will make the fasting time frames considerably less demanding to traverse.

2. **Fast overnight**. Toss yourself a bone and aim at fasting as the night progressed, so that you are (ideally) dozing amid at least eight hours.

3. **Rewire your way of thinking**. Consider fasting as taking a break from the consumption of food, not as a time of deprivation. It can be an approach to breaking away from the repetitiveness of agonizing over (a) when you have to eat next and (b) what to eat. This is the mentality that will permit you to take after a fasting arrangement long haul.

4. **Overcommit**. It might appear to be strange. However, the best arrangement is regularly to begin when you're occupied — not on a day when you will be perched on the coach desiring to eat a snack.

5. **Hit the exercise center**. Integrating intermittent fasting with steady practice will assist you to get awesome results. The exercises do not need to be hardcore or insane; it can be something as basic as a full-body strength exercising routine a few times each week.

Benefits of Intermittent Fasting

Fasting's most evident advantage is weight reduction. Though, there are a bunch of benefits past this, a considerable lot of which were known in the old days. The fasting time frames were regularly called 'purification,' 'cleanses' or 'detoxifications,' yet the thought is the same – to refrain from eating for some time for reasons related to health.

Individuals envisioned that this duration from sustenance would clear their bodies' frameworks of toxins. They were more right than they knew. In this chapter we explain what the physical benefits of intermittent fasting are.

Decreasing Weight & Body Fats

Studies have demonstrated that intermittent fasting is related to weight reduction. While a significant number of the patients are more worried about the general decrease in weight, likewise there is a lot of patients who need to put on weight, particularly fit body weight or bulk.

Furthermore, some of these patients express worry that intermittent fasting may prompt to a reduction in muscle mass. Luckily, studies have proven that intermittent fasting causes a positive move on digestion that preserves muscle.

Here is the reason: Amid the most widely recognized fasting length of around 18 to 24 hours, the body cells move from utilizing glucose as their essential fuel source to utilizing fat. This implies our fat stores, in particular, triglycerides, are broken down and utilized for vitality. Until the third day of fasting is when the breakdown of proteins for fuel starts. Hence, intermittent fasting remains a possibility for improving health, even in those people needing to keep up their energy or pick up some extra muscle mass.

Without going into a lot of the science in this matter, the shift on digestion from glucose to fat might be most articulated after around 18 hours of fasting, recommending potential advantages from occasional entire day fasts. This would suggest that a method like *Leangains* would be more effective, although this cannot be proven completely.

Improved Cardiovascular Disease Risk Profile

Intermittent fasting leads to a decrease of aggregate cholesterol by around 20%. This turns out to be significantly more noteworthy when we take a look at the breakdown of the impacts on High-Density Lipoprotein (HDL), triglycerides, and Low-Density Lipoprotein (LDL). This might become a little bit technical, so read closely and regularly refer to the terminology below.

Below is a simplification of theses terminologies:

- Triglycerides are a kind of fat used to store abundance energy from our eating regimen, and high ranks might be related to cardiovascular sickness and insulin resistance (we need low levels of triglycerides); Triglycerides is the bad stuff.
- LDL is the "terrible cholesterol" (the most noticeably bad are little, thick LDL, and the less hostile form is huge, fluffy LDL); LDL is the bad stuff.
- HDL is the "great cholesterol" (we would prefer not to see HDL diminish, and regularly we would lean toward it increment); HDL is the good stuff.

Since the aggregate cholesterol on a blood board is gotten from a recipe including LDL, HDL, and triglycerides, we need to ensure that abatement in cholesterol originates from diminishments in LDL or triglycerides, and not brought down HDL.

Here is what happens to cholesterol with intermittent fasting. Not exclusively does LDL diminish by around 25% following two months on another day by day quick, yet surprisingly better, we observe a decline in little LDL particles. Furthermore, reminisce, little, thick LDL particles are related to an expanded danger of cardiovascular illness when contrasted and an equivalent number of huge, fluffy LDL particles.

Note: Little, thick LDL is best seen as an intermediary for LDL molecule number, which is a more noteworthy hazard consider for coronary illness than aggregate or LDL cholesterol.

Thus, intermittent fasting positively moves LDL both by diminishing aggregate LDL and furthermore by diminishing the little, thick LDL particles. We additionally observe a decrement in triglycerides by as much as 32% beneath levels measured before executing intermittent fasting. That's a good thing. Also, with intermittent fasting, there is no bad impact on HDL.

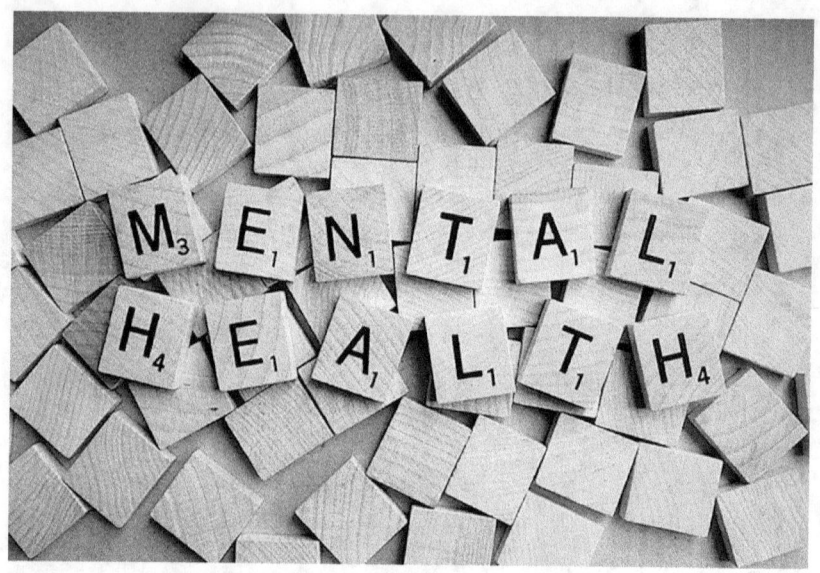

Improved Mental Health

Intermittent fasting is related to enhanced brain coordination and learning reaction and abatement in oxidative anxiety (consider oxidative worry as what we regularly consider "ordinary" age-related change).

In this way, fasting may enhance health aging of the mind and abatement the intellectual deterioration that is, for the most part, considered an ordinary piece of growing old.

Reductions in Neuro-Inflammation

Interminable neuro-inflammation is progressively connected with neurodegenerative diseases like Alzheimer's and mood disorders, for example, depression. Many people suffer from some type of inflammation problem. Studies have shown that intermittent fasting changes the gene expression to consider a versatile response.

Fasting may have a helpful part in conditions related with inflammation. If you wish to learn more about this, I wrote an entire book on this topic, titled: "Anti-Inflammatory Diet". More details can be found at the end of this book.

Benefits Regulation of Hormones

The impacts of fasting on hormones are multi-faceted. Fasting dramatically affects human development hormone levels. Expanded HGH brings about more noteworthy endurance with speedier muscle repair and development and also slowing down the process of growing old. One review demonstrated that interim exercising while fasting improved HGH by 1300% in ladies and 2000% in gentlemen.

Important to every one of us is the effect of fasting on the levels of insulin. Insulin resistance – when cells overlook insulin as it rings the entryway chime attempting to convey its bundle of energy (glucose) – is an essential contributing component related to about each chronic ailment. Fasting, particularly when integrated with exercise, is a standout amongst the best methods for the normalizing sensitivity of insulin.

Leptin, the hormone that controls the storage of fat and also hunger signs, and ghrelin, another hormone that tells your mind the body is hungry, are likewise standardized by routine fasting.

Fat cells normally produce leptin, and it works by instructing the mind to switch off hunger signals when levels of body fats are adequate for survival and propagation. Since fat is fundamental for survival, leptin is a piece of the reason low-fat diets never work and typically just outcomes to the individual feeling hungry every single moment. Curiously, high levels of leptin have been witnessed in overweight individuals, yet few who battle with weight will disclose to you they seldom feel hungry. The body is hollering at the mind to quit eating yet the cerebrum has turned out to be deaf to the signs. This occurs by a similar component that prompts to insulin resistance: steady overexposure to large amounts of the hormone.

Fasting, and specifically when joined with reduced sugar ingestion, permits the mind to wipe out its ears and appropriately hear leptin calling.

Detoxification

In spite of what numerous item manufacturers would have you think, purifying and detoxifying is something your body constantly does, and it is going on 24 hours a day. A large number of cellular procedures that happen each day inflicts significant damage on individual cells, especially on the mitochondria.

In a perfect world, the body distinguishes these worn out parts of cells and replaces them (a procedure usually alluded to as autophagy). This is a consistent duty. While this procedure is programmed and continuous, it can be essentially thwarted by a terrible diet.

Even worse, it can even be impeded by a sound diet. Just by the way that when your body is processing incoming food, it diminishes its cell custodial obligations. Giving your body time to concentrate exclusively on the repair of cells can be unbelievably helpful for ideal cleansing.

Intriguing research has turned out on the advantages of fasting on neuron driven sicknesses like Huntington's and Alzheimer's. As autophagy is expanded amid a fasting state rundown mitochondria and other molecules are destroyed from the neurons. You can see the association then between the amplified detoxification capacities while fasting and a reduced process of aging. This is profound cleansing in its most genuine form. Indeed, intermittent fasting might be the ultimate (natural) body detox procedure you can think of. Goodbye detox diets.

Practical Benefits of Fasting

Fasting offers numerous critical one-of-a-kind advantages that are not accessible in ordinary diets. Where diets confound life, fasting makes it simpler. Where weight diets are costly, fasting is free. Where diets can require some serious time, fasting saves time.

Where diets are restricted, fasting is accessible anyplace. Where diets have variable adequacy, fasting has unchallenged efficacy. There is not any more intense strategy for bringing down the insulin level and reducing body weight. But there's much more to the benefits.

The Seven Practical Benefits of Fasting

Low-carb high-fat (LCHF) eating regimens are without a doubt efficient for weight reduction, yet we can improve by including intermittent fasting, which provides a lot of advantages not offered by conventional dieting. Both eating methodologies have a similar objective, which is to reduce the impact of insulin.

While a large number of people believe that calories cause a gain of weight, which is a myth. Insulin is the principal driver of the increase in weight.

LCHF diets bring down insulin instead of calories and in this way are successful weight reduction diets. However, fasting shows improvement over LCHF so the two might be integrated for most extreme impact. Here are my main seven focal points of fasting. We will start with number 7 and count down from there.

No.#7: Simplicity

LCHF diets are not simple for individuals to get it. Numerous foodstuffs contain concealed high-caloric sugars in the list of ingredients. Individuals may not comprehend the contrasts between sugars, fats, and proteins.

To make it considerably more mind boggling, starch vary in their fattening potential. What about fiber? What about the idea of net carbs? What about starch that is resistant? The inquiries are unending. It is sufficiently troublesome for a knowledgeable English-talking, computer literate individual to embrace a strict LCHF diet. That, as well as there is all that clashing advice flying around the net and the wireless transmissions.

The low-fat eating routine has been inculcated into individuals throughout the previous forty years, so they it was hard to incorporate loads of natural and healthy fats into their diets. A unique approach, for example, fasting is significantly easier for individuals to get it.

Fasting is very simple to the point that it can be clarified in only two sentences. Eat nothing including sugars or sweeteners. Drink Coffee, water, tea or bone soup. That is it. Indeed, even with this basic strategy, understanding the complexities can take hours of clarifications.

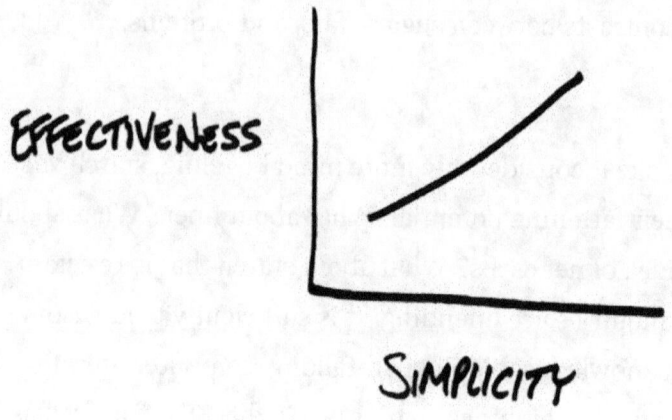

EFFECTIVENESS

SIMPLICITY

The most evident advantage to effortlessness though is exhibited by the startlingly basic diagram above. The less difficult, the more effective. And obviously, fasting is as simple as it gets.

No.#6: Price

It is highly recommended that individual eat natural, local grass consumed meat and stay away from the white bread and food that is processed, actually these foods are regularly ten times the cost. A few people can't afford to eat that well.

This is because of the bending impact of government subsidies on the cost of foodstuffs. Since grains appreciate considerable government endowments, it is far less expensive to make something out of flour than entire whole foods. Sustaining a family on a financial plan is a considerable simpler when you purchase white bread and pasta.

In any case, that does not mean they ought to be destined to a lifetime of sort two diabetes and inability. Fasting is completely free. It is not just free, but rather it helps an individual to save cash since one does not have to purchase any food staffs. Nothing beats free, aside from, obviously, sparing cash. Who cannot utilize a couple of additional dollars in their pocket while shedding pounds and improving health-wise in the meantime? It is as if you are being paid to shed some pounds!

No.#5: Convenience

Eating a home cooked starch meal is fabulous. However, there are many individuals who essentially don't have sufficient time or desire to do as such. The number of meals consumed away from people's houses has been exponentially rising in the course of recent decades.

While there are numerous individuals who attempt to bolster the 'slow food' locomotion, it is evident that they are battling a losing fight.

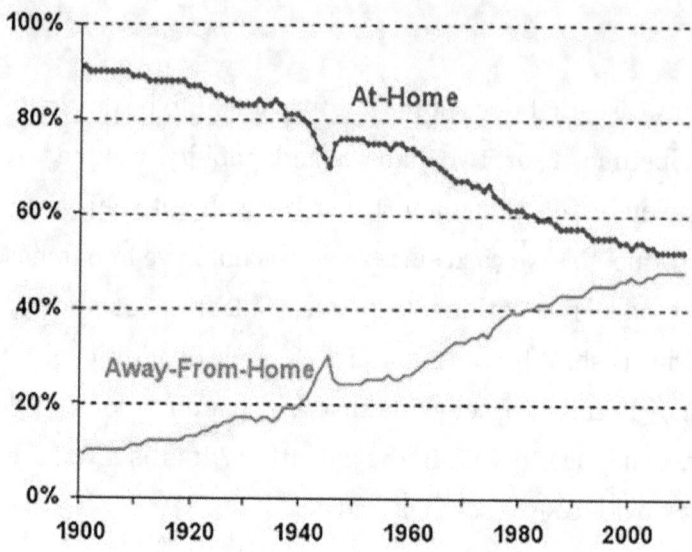

Requesting that individuals dedicate themselves to home cooking, as respectable as it might be, is not a triumphant methodology. Fasting, then again is the inverse. You spare time since there is no time spent purchasing food staffs, preparing the food and cleaning. It is an approach to rearranging your life in a simpler manner. For instance, if you do not take breakfast you can spare a lot of time and furthermore cash.

Where numerous diets entangle your life (eat this, however not that, and just a tad bit of the other), fasting makes your life simpler it. Spare time and spare cash? It simply does not get any swifter.

No.#4: Cheat Days

It is not good to encourage individuals to never, until kingdom come, feed on ice cream or any form of dessert. Of course, you may have the capacity to swear off of it for six months, or 1 year, however forever? What's more, would you truly desire to? Contemplate about it. Consider the delight of relishing a particularly tasty pastry at a wedding feast.

Do we have to deny ourselves that tad bit of delight until the end of time? Give every single person of us a chance to make the most of our birthday serving of salad! Thanksgiving kale celebration! Yeah, life just got somewhat less sparkly. Forever is quite a while.

You cannot consume dessert each and every day, except fasting gives you the capacity to sometimes appreciate that treat when you are in party or dining with friends, you can adjust the scales by fasting. After all, this is the cycle of life. "Cheat" days are critical because they create compliance for alternate days. It makes the eating regimen simpler to take after and transforms it into a way of life. An essential part of fasting is to ensure that it fits into your life.

Everybody experiences great days and awful days. There are celebrating days and dreadful days, and that is life. Your diet additionally should be intermittent. There are times to eat a ton and celebrate. However, there similarly should be days where you fast, to compensate for it. It is, however, keen to mention that cheat days are not recommended if an individual has an obsession with a certain kind of food or sugar. Similar to like the situation where cheat days are not suggested for alcoholics.

No.#3: Power

It is difficult to lose weight. Everyone realizes that. The most critical question of any dietary intercession is this – will it work? The caloric decrement diet sounds like it ought to work, yet does it work? The appropriate response is, most of the time, no.

For some individuals, certain diets normally work excellently, however, flop absolutely for others. Some of the time, diets work for a certain time frame, and afterward appear to slow down. Alone among dietary intercessions, fasting is all around powerful, since it is the speediest and most effective approach for reduction of insulin. It moreover contains practically boundless power. What do I mean? A few eating regimens have just 1 "power" setting.

On the off chance that you take after the Mediterranean eating routine, yet you are unable to shed pounds, then what? How would you turn out to be more 'Mediterranean'? It's unthinkable. There is just a single power setting, and it either works, or it does not. But when you come to fasting, this is not the case. You can essentially keep fasting until the weight you want is shaded. Therefore there is boundless power.

No.#2: Flexibility

Fasting should be possible whenever and in wherever. Just in case you don't feel well for any reason, you stop. It is completely reversible inside minutes. Consider bariatric surgery (stomach stapling). These surgeries are performed as such that individuals can fast for prolonged timeframes.

What's more is that they tend to work but for a short time. However, these surgeries have huge amounts of difficulties, nearly all of which are irreversible.

There is no set term. You can fast for 16 hours or even 16 days. There is no set timetable. You can fast a considerable measure this week and none one week from now. It can be adjusted depending on your schedule. You can fast for any reason or no reason whatsoever. Besides, why might we make an assumption that someone can't fast for one week or 1 month while never having attempted it?

No.#1: Add to Any Diet

Here is the greatest benefit of all. Fasting can be included to whichever diet you prefer. That is on account of fasting is not something you do, but rather something you do not do. It is subtraction as opposed to addition. And eating pattern instead of the avoidance of certain foods.

It is quite simple to use fasting as an addition to dieting, simply because it is so easy to do. Fasting saves cash. Fasting also saves time. It is adaptable, effective. Accessible whenever, anyplace. What could be superior to that?

Practical Tips for Fasting

In the past, when religious fasting was a communal undertaking, these kinds of tips were passed on from era to era. If not, companions would regularly have valuable exhortation on the best way to deal with the fasting, since there are unquestionably a few issues that usually emerge. Be that as it may, with the decrease in the act of fasting, these sorts of exhortation are regularly hard to get; unless you're perusing this.

There is a wide range of guidelines for fasting. For instance, fasting is honed from dawn to nightfall, and no refreshments or foods are taken during the Ramadan. Different sorts of fasting will just confine certain kinds of foods – for instance, keeping away from meat for 24 hours. However, it is most likely you are not fasting for religious purposes when you picked up this book. So there is no set in stone principles to go by. Fasting that is recommended for the reduction of weight and health is mostly adaptable to your personal situation. There are a few recommendations that can help you create that optimal situation for yourself.

Water

All refreshments and foods that contain calories are withheld for the period of fasting. Staying hydrated all through the fast is highly recommended. Water, both still and shimmering, is dependably a decent decision.

Intend to drink approximately two liters of water day by day. As a decent practice, begin each day with seven ounces of cool water to guarantee sufficient hydration as the day starts. Include a crush of lemon or lime to the water just in case add some flavor to it, in case you wish. On the other hand, you can include a few cuts of cucumber or orange to a pitcher of water, so ass to add some flavor, and after that relish the water for the remaining duration of the day. Nonetheless, manufactured flavors or sweeteners are disallowed. Crystal Light, Tang or Kool-Aid ought not to be added to the water that you will be drinking while you are practicing intermittent fasting.

Tea

There are many types of tea, and all are incredible, including green, dark, oolong and herbal. Teas can frequently be mixed with the assortment and can be appreciated hot or frosty. To add flavor to your tea, you can utilize various spices, for example, cinnamon or nutmeg.

It is likewise acceptable to including a little measure of milk or cream (regardless of the possibility that it is, in fact, a small cheat). Milk is a great enhancer of flavor that is acceptable to use when fasting. Non-natural sweeteners, flavors or sugar are **not** permitted. The *catechins* in green tea are alleged to help smother hunger, and thus green tea is highly recommended.

Coffee

Coffee, decaffeinated or caffeinated, is likewise allowed. A little measure of cream or milk is suitable, despite the fact that these do contain a few calories. Flavors, for example, sweeteners, sugar or non-natural flavors are not acceptable, but cinnamon may be added to the coffee.

Iced coffee is an incredible selection particularly on days that temperatures are above the normal. Coffee likely has numerous medical advantages.

Bone Broth

The bone broth that is homemade, produced using hamburger, pork, chicken or fish bones, is a decent selection for days that you are fasting. Another appropriate option is vegetable juices; even though the bone broth has more supplements than it. Including a decent squeeze of sea salt to the soup will assist you to remain hydrated.

Alternate liquids — tea, water, and coffee — don't contain sodium, so throughout longer fasting periods, it is conceivable to wind up distinctly salt-drained. There is far more serious threat in getting to be distinctly salt depleted throughout fasting, even if many dread the additional sodium. For shorter fasts, for example, the 24-and 36-hour type, additional sodium is not needed, but rather throughout longer fasts it can be essential.

All vegetables, herbs or flavors are extraordinary add-ons to soup; yet in a perfect world do not include bouillon cubes, which are loaded with manufactured flavors and monosodium glutamate. Be careful with canned broths: they are poor replications of the broths that are homemade.

Break Your Fast Gently

Be mindful so as to break your fast delicately. There is a characteristic inclination to eat a lot of food when you have completed your fast. Strangely, the vast majority do not portray overwhelming appetite, yet all the more a mental desire to eat food.

Stomach discomfort might be prompted by overeating immediately after completing the fast. While not genuine, it can be very uncomfortable. This issue has a tendency to be self-correcting, that is, the vast majority will dodge it next time.

Have a go at breaking your fast with a modest bunch of nuts or a little serving of salad to begin. At that point sit tight for a quarter to half an hour. This will ordinarily give time for any rushes of hunger to pass, and permit you to adjust progressively. Apples are also great to eat after longer fasting periods.

Brief term fasts (less than 24 hours) for the most part require no extraordinary breaking of the fast.

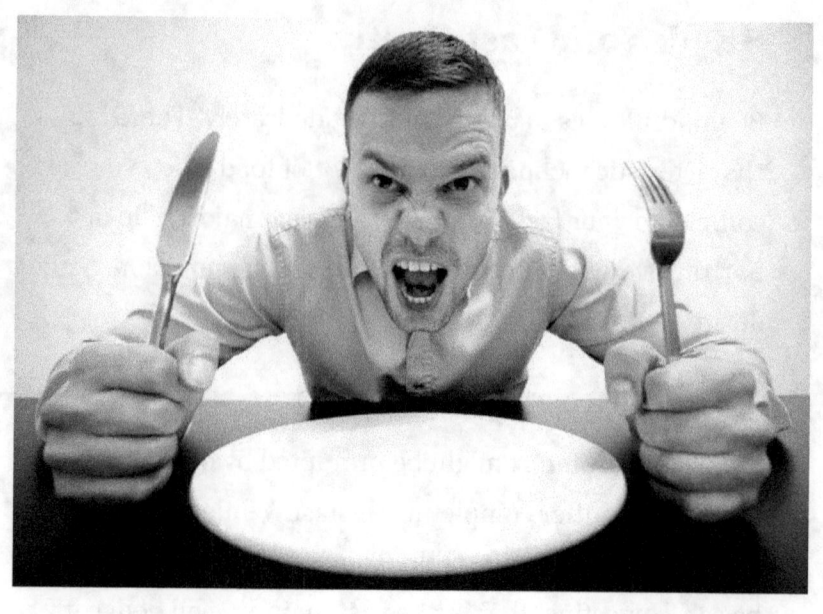

What to Do When You Get Hungry

This is presumably the main concern for most people. You are likely to expect that hunger will overwhelm you, and you will not be able to control yourself. The fact is that hunger does not persevere, but rather comes in waves. In case you're encountering hunger, it will pass. Remaining occupied with something throughout the day that you are fasting is normally helpful. Drink green tea when your stomach hurts a lot. Fasting when you are having a bustling day at work keeps your brain off eating.

Your hunger will be repressed as the body become used to fasting, since it will begin to burn the fat that is stored. Many individuals take note that as they fast, hunger does not upsurge but instead begins to diminish. This is why the starting phase is often perceived as the toughest. There are natural things that can help smother hunger. Here are the main five normal hunger suppressants:

1. **Water:** As specified sometime recently, begin your day with a full glass of frosty water. Remaining hydrated counteracts hunger. Drinking a glass of water preceding a feast may likewise lessen hunger. Sparkling mineral water may assist for loud stomachs and cramping.

2. **Chia Seeds:** Chia seeds are high in dissolvable fiber and omega three fatty acids. These seeds take in water and form a gel when absorbed fluid for half an hour, which may help in the suppression hunger. These seeds can be taken dry or made into a gel or pudding.

3. **Coffee:** While many accept that caffeine stifles hunger, studies demonstrate that this impact could be identified with antioxidants. Both general coffee and decaffeinated indicates greater appetite concealment than caffeine in water. Given its presumable medical advantages, there is no motivation to restraining coffee admission. The caffeine that is in the coffee may

likewise raise your metabolism and thus boost the burning of fat.

4. **Cinnamon:** Studies have shown that cinnamon assists in the suppression of hunger and are also slowing the emptying of gastric. It might likewise help in bringing down blood sugars and subsequently valuable in weight reduction. Cinnamon might be added to coffee and all types of teas for a delectable change.

5. **Green tea:** Full of polyphenols and anti-oxidants, green tea is an awesome guide for dieters. The strong anti-oxidants may assist to inspire weight reduction and metabolism.

Exercise While Fasting

A wide range of activity, including resistance (weights) and cardio, are recommended. There is a typical misperception that eating is important to supply "vitality" to the functioning body. That is not valid. Energy is supplied by the liver via *gluconeogenesis*. This is process of delivering energy to the body. Amid longer fasting periods, the muscles are additionally ready to utilize unsaturated fats straightforwardly for energy. Your body will not eat muscle mass (unless you take fasting to the extreme and dangerous regions).

Fasting is a perfect time to work out, since your levels of adrenaline will be higher. The increase in development hormone that accompanies fasting may likewise even cause muscle development.

These points of interest have driven numerous people, particularly those inside the working out group, to take a more noteworthy enthusiasm for purposely working out in the fasted state. People with diabetes who are taking prescriptive drugs, nevertheless, must play it safe since they may encounter low blood sugars for the period of exercise and fasting. Always consult a dietician before fasting when you are suffering from a chronic disease like diabetes.

Is Intermittent Fasting For Everybody?

While intermittent fasting works for some people, it is not a solid match for everyone. It's quite tough for some people to go on a period of fasting. And for people who suffer from any type of chronic ailment, it's advisable to not partake in any fasting at all, as it may harm your health.

Above all else, Intermittent fasting is not simply one more method for saying "free ride." Keeping on eating a diet high in foods that are processed while randomly skipping meals will not assist you to enhance your health or shed some fats. Some will discover intermittent fasting is tiresome or even bothersome, making it impossible to rehearse. What is more, for others, its dangers far exceed any potential advantages. Truth be told, for a few people intermittent fasting could be out and out risky. You presumably need to know whether you fall into that classification before you avoid your next meal. Let's use the metaphor of a traffic light to see if you're good to go.

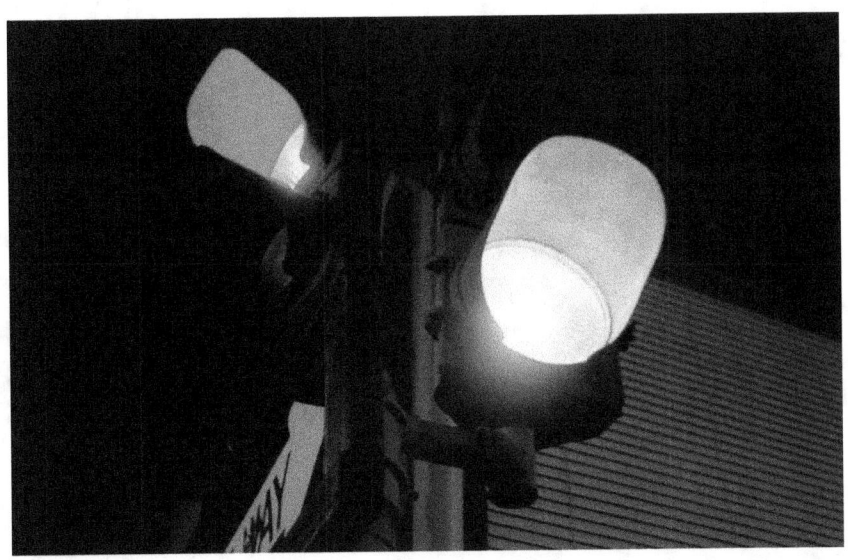

Green Light: When you're Safe

As far as studies have shown, a person is destined to be effective with discontinuous fasting if:

- You have a background marked by observing calorie and food consumption (e.g., you've "counted calories" sometime recently)
- You have already established yourself as a frequent exerciser
- You are living alone, and you are single, or you do not have youngsters
- Your lover (on the off chance that you have one) is greatly supportive

- Your employment permits you to have times where your performance is not up to standard while you adjust to another arrangement
- You are male with strong health and physique

The initial five variables will permit you to incorporate the conventions with your way of life all the more effectively, while the last condition (being male) appears to influence men about intermittent fasting.

Yellow Light: When to Be Cautious

In the meantime, in case you meet the accompanying criteria, you might need to continue with precaution:

- You have children, or you are married and often dine with family
- You have a job that is performance oriented or a customer confronting occupation
- You are an athlete, or you indulge in sports
- You're female

The initial three conditions make it substantially harder to take after intermittent fasting conventions and may make it unfeasible for you. Likewise, attempting to fast, may clash with execution objectives for your sport.

On the last condition, a few experimenters propose that for ladies, fasting causes restlessness, nervousness, sporadic periods, and different signs of hormone dysregulation. Specifically, ladies appear to not do better on the stricter fasting methods, compared to males. So in case you are female, and you want to have a go at intermittent fasting, I suggest starting with an exceptionally relaxed approach.

Red Light: When to Avoid

At long last, there are a few people who truly should not attempt practicing IF by any stretch of the imagination. Try not to attempt it if:

- You are pregnant
- You have a background marked by disordered eating
- You are stressed a lot
- You don't rest soundly
- You're new to exercise and diet
- You have hormonal imbalances (mostly in females)

In case you're new to eating regimen and exercise, intermittent fasting may resemble an enchantment slug for the reduction of weight. In any case, you would be a great deal more brilliant to deal with any nutrition deficiencies before you begin exploring different avenues regarding fasting. First, make certain you are beginning from a strong nutritious stage.

Ladies who are pregnant have additional energy needs; therefore in case you are beginning a family, this is not an opportunity to fast. Likewise in case, you are under serious stress as well as not dozing. Your body does not need additional stress but more energy. Furthermore, in case you have battled with any eating disorder before, you most likely perceive that a fasting convention could lead you down a way that may make advance issues for you. Why disturb your health? You can accomplish comparative advantages in different ways.

Side Effects of Fasting Diets

Obviously, it's not all sunshine and butterflies when you're trying out new ways of dieting. Fasting is no exception to that rule, as it does have a multitude of different side-effects. This chapter discusses the most prominent ones people experience during a period of intermittent fasting. So keep this in mind when you are attempting to start with fasting yourself.

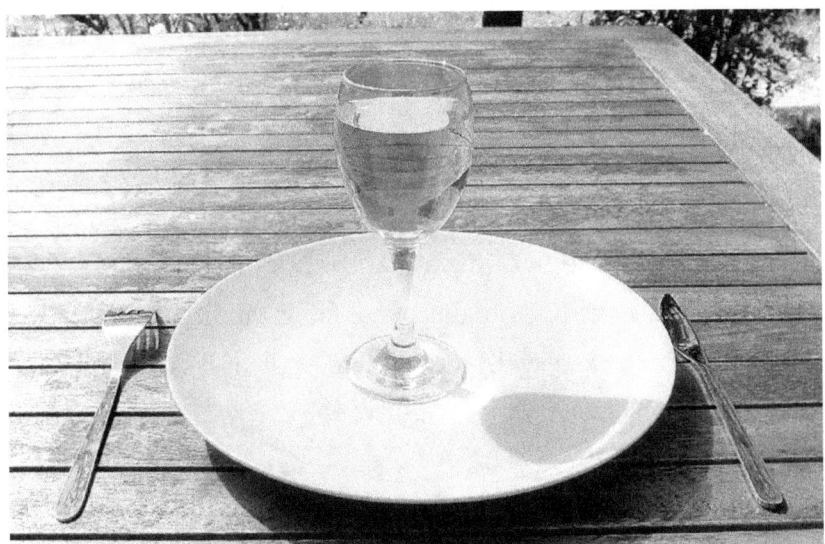

Could Cause Common Dietary Issues

Individuals seldom talk about this, however at its most extreme, irregular fasting's 'gorge then vomit'-mindset could trigger or worsen bulimia and other dietary issues. The *anything goes* attitude a few specialists allow throughout the eating state could propel somebody to overeat, guilt creation, disgrace, and different issues that exclusive turn out to be more regrettable after some time. For somebody with mental dietary issues or emotional disorders, intermittent fasting has the capability of amplifying these problems.

You Might Increase Cortisol Levels

Skipping dinners increase your anxiety hormone cortisol, which I consider a dark master of metabolism. "From an evolutionary point of view, that fleeting rise was a win since it got the body to discharge fat as vitality. Ladies appear to be especially susceptible to the risks of fasting.

This has the capability of keeping cortisol elevated when it ought to decrease and make the undesired impact of putting away fat and breaking muscles down. Have you been around intermittent fasters? Dreadful to be around!"

Undesirable Obsession with Food

For instance, let's consider that you have been fasting throughout the morning, your colleague opens her broccoli chicken Chinese takeaway during lunch hour, and all of a sudden whatever you can consider is the thing that you will feed on to break your fast during suppertime.

Hunger demonstrates an intense, transformative system that held us alive once upon a time. With our present day omnipresent bodegas and goodies machines, craving isn't regularly an issue, and we infrequently face it. The issue is everything else takes a backseat to eating at the point at which you are starving. With intermittent fasting, that could turn into an obsession with rationally arranging your next meal. Everything gets to be distinctly about eating your food.

Overdependence on Coffee

Most intermittent fasting arrangements permit caffeine, a stimulant that can prop you up for quite a long time when you are not feeding on anything. When you are fasting, you may wind up inclining toward coffeehouses all the more regularly to get your settle that ensures you are still pressing on without food.

Particularly for moderate metabolizers, that third mug of black roast could cut into your rest cycle. It is an endless loop, as caffeine can upset sleep and encourage melancholy and nervousness. Coffee additionally amps up cortisol, which is the body's stress hormone. Cortisol's key task is to elevate the levels of glucose. Indeed, even little increments in cortisol, for example, those accomplished when drinking caffeine, can elevate glucose level and raise insulin resistance.

Inflammation & Food Intolerance

Fasting makes you hungry, generating a free-for-all jump into profound dish pizza and a hot fudge sundae when you eat. Do not worry about it that a noteworthy caloric over-burden and glucose spike and crash that at last prompt to more yearnings.

Your "break the fast" dish will probably contain gluten, dairy, and other potential responsive sustenances — maybe in huge sums — that add to leaky gut, facilitating food intolerance, Candida, and other gut problems, and amplified inflammation.

Decreases Athletic Performance

It's alright to work out decently when fasting. In any case, doing extraordinary exercises like power-lifting, cross-fit or high-intensity interim exercising can harm you. Research indicates that athletic execution as a fact lessens when fasting. Different reviews likewise demonstrate increment of exhaustion after exceptional exercises when fasting. Either way, I don't tell you to hit the gym during intermittent fasting because I want you to suffer. It's simply to keep your original strength up, and to avoid you become something that resembles a wet noodle (just joking, obviously), in the long run.

Heartburn

Many individuals encounter acid reflux while doing intermittent fasting. Now and then the acid reflux corrects itself between a month and one and a half months, however just in case they do not, then you ought to see a specialist. The body discharges acids at specific times since it was used to the old eating patterns and thus causes the heartburn. What's more, when you change the eating design, it will attempt to stick to past eating practices.

Headaches

Cerebral pains are a typical event when fasting. Most people grumble of mild migraines from time to time while others encounter them all through the fasting period. Drinking enough water alleviates the annoying headaches to some degree. However, drinking tea or other hot beverages will often help you out with this nuisance even better.

Affects Pregnant Women Negatively

A few studies have proven that fasting amid pregnancy does not influence the unborn child or the mother. In any case, you might need to abstain from intermittent fasting while pregnant. Give hunger a chance to direct what you eat when in this period. Try not to famish yourself or the baby for the sake of fasting. All things considered, fasting might not be of advantageous during pregnancy. Truth be told, the Intermittent Fasting negative effects on this list can make life difficult for you when pregnant.

Frequent Diarrhea

Numerous intermittent fasting PR specialists encounter diarrhea in the wake of fasting. However, how extreme it can be, relies on upon to what extent the fast was. Longer fasting span causes dangerous diarrhea. This is brought about by high liquid intake – drinking a considerable measure of water and coffee.

Brain Fog

Mind mist and feeling slow are additionally normal with numerous intermittent fasting dieters. In any case, the brain fog after some time normally goes away. Truth be told, it is a fact that fasting that is long term enhances cerebrum function.

Affects Hormones in Women Negatively

A few ladies who attempt Intermittent Fasting claim to go through missed periods, unsettling metabolic influences and early-onset menopause.

Ladies' hormones used in reproduction are profoundly sensitively to vitality admission. Therefore going for extended periods without nourishment influences how these hormones function.

Low Energy

One of the paramount worries for people who need to attempt Intermittent Fasting is low energy. What's more, it's an honest concern. Low energy and general weakness are as a result of intermittent fasting. This can prevent you from working out or remaining active physically.

Fasting Best Practices

In case you're a busy person, work 50 or more hours in seven days, and invest the greater part of your free time moving children around and working the honey-do list, exercising day-by-day and eating healthy might be a challenge. So avoiding a couple of meals and resembling the Men's Health cover model may sound truly engaging. But not jump to conclusions so quick. You cannot simply skip some meals and get amazing outcomes.

Keep in mind, some of these types of fasts take after particular conventions. Simply eating randomly and after that not eating is the thing that gets many individuals overweight in any case. However, in case you are enthusiastic about attempting intermittent fasting, here are some things that you should first consider:

1. **Choices on which food to take matter**. Because you are not frequently eating does not mean the fundamental guidelines of good nutrition do not matter. A 20 hour fast and after that burning through 4 hours eating junk food stuff will not get you lean. You have to concentrate on great sources of carbohydrates, solid fats, protein, and heaps of fruits and veggies.

2. **Be patient**. In case you are a major fan of breakfast, fasting will be a key trial of willpower–especially for an initial couple of weeks. However, here is the great part. It gets better–much better–after 14 days or somewhere in the vicinity. Stick it out. You're not kicking the bucket –you're quite recently hungry.

3. **Working out makes a difference**. The best fasting conventions should have you hit the gym. It is healthier and efficient to practice while doing intermittent fasting.

4. **Timing is everything; it is however not the only thing.** Knowing the period you are required to fast and breaking the fast with a major meal is recommended but also do not forget to work out so as to achieve the desired results.

5. **Progress slowly**. It's vital, to begin with, the trial fast and permit yourself to get "excellent at it" before progressing to more regular or complex fasting conventions. Many encounters are going only a couple of hours without eating unendurable. It requires determination and practice. Therefore patience is required. Overwhelm the simple strides before moving further up the fasting ladder.

6. **Do not overdo intermittent fasting**. After accomplishing awesome outcomes with week by week fast, do not multiply the frequency of fasting so as to get a double result. It might not work for you.

7. **It's as yet a way of life**. There are no eating regimens, just ways of life. What's more, any eating routine that you were unable to follow theoretically take after.

8. **Some should not do intermittent fasting.** Anybody and everybody ought to try the trial fast. It is factual that you get to understand a lot about oneself when you abandon food for an entire day. As deliberated earlier, there are various categories of people that should practice intermittent fasting and those who should not even think about it. We already discussed some risk-prone groups earlier on. If you are included in those groups, don't fast.

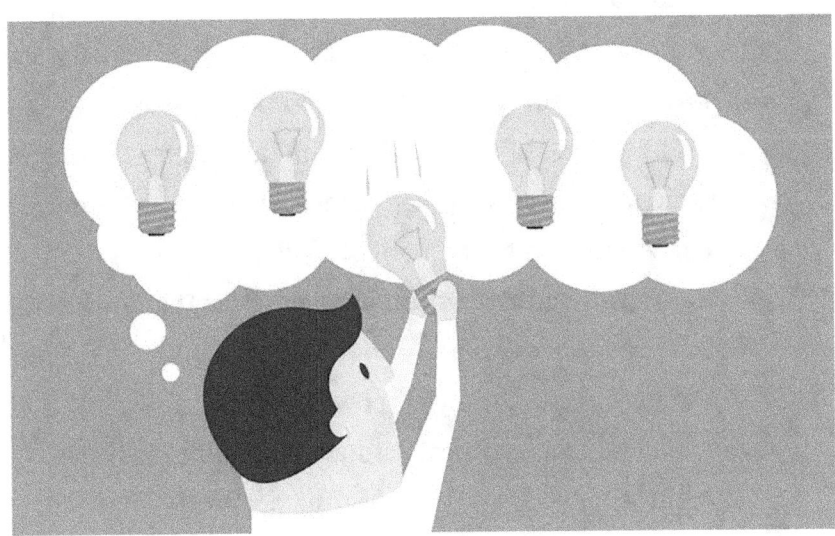

Remember the Basics

One extra thing. Always remember that there is no enchantment pill (or enchantment eating arrangement), and when all is said and done, grasping the essentials is as yet your best tactic. Here are the basics, clearly outlined.

1. **Eating food that is of great quality**. Fresh and natural food that its nutrient density is high is very essential, paying little respect to the eating style. Therefore settle on the best decisions you can manage and make awareness of food a priority.
2. **Slow eating**. Hurrying through meals negatively affects digestion and befuddles satiety centers in the cerebrum. Therefore take it slow. It assists control intake and enhances your satisfaction in eating.
3. **Eating sensible portions**. At the point when calories are controlled, significant development is made. Overeating is as yet probable with intermittent fasting, similarly as it is with each other eating pattern. Simply concentrate on the amount of food.
4. **Consuming food when you are hungry, and not eating when you are most certainly not**. Figuring out how to tune into your craving and listen to your actual hunger is critical. Utilizing mindfulness when eating is a best practice for eating healthy.
5. **Working out frequently.** Obviously, working out and adhering to a good diet are two sides of a similar

coin. They both assist in promoting good health and a fit body however in various ways. So utilize both.

How to Begin

Since you know every single of the basics of fasting, how would you begin? You simply adhere to these steps:

- **Choose** your preferred method of intermittent fasting;
- Settle for the **timeframe** you need or wish to fast;
- **Begin** fasting. In case you don't feel well, or in case you have any worries, then stop and look for assistance;
- Proceed with all your typical **exercises** outside of eating. Remain occupied and live regularly. Envision you are "eating" a meal of your fat;
- Break the fasting **softly** and steadily;
- **Repeat** the process until you achieve results, combine with other diets if needed.

Yes. It truly is THAT straightforward. With some effort, your enthusiasm for intermittent fasting will increase, and your body will adapt to all the changes. It's that little starting period in between where most of the nuisances and suffering is. Beat that though start, and you're well on your way to a great revolution in your personal diet plan!

Parting Words

Intermittent fasting can be valuable for some individuals, enhancing their concentration and vitality, and making weight control a more cognizant determination. Nonetheless, it is unquestionably not for everyone, as we discovered in the chapters discussed in this book. Just in case you are keen on giving it a shot, it is recommended that you pick the type of intermittent fasting that impacts you and your objectives, and test it.

Give it an opportunity to adjust. Lest you have never fasted, it might take a short time to get accustomed to it. At that point evaluate your results. In case you did, incredible! Just in case you didn't, do not get stressed up. There are a lot of different patterns of eating accessible that might fit better with your one of a kind desire. If you wish to learn more about balancing the body using food as a tool, I highly recommend you to check out some of my other books. If you suffer from the common nuisance known as inflammation (a subject we briefly touched upon in this book), I warmly invite you to check out my other recently released book, titled "Anti-Inflammatory Diet".

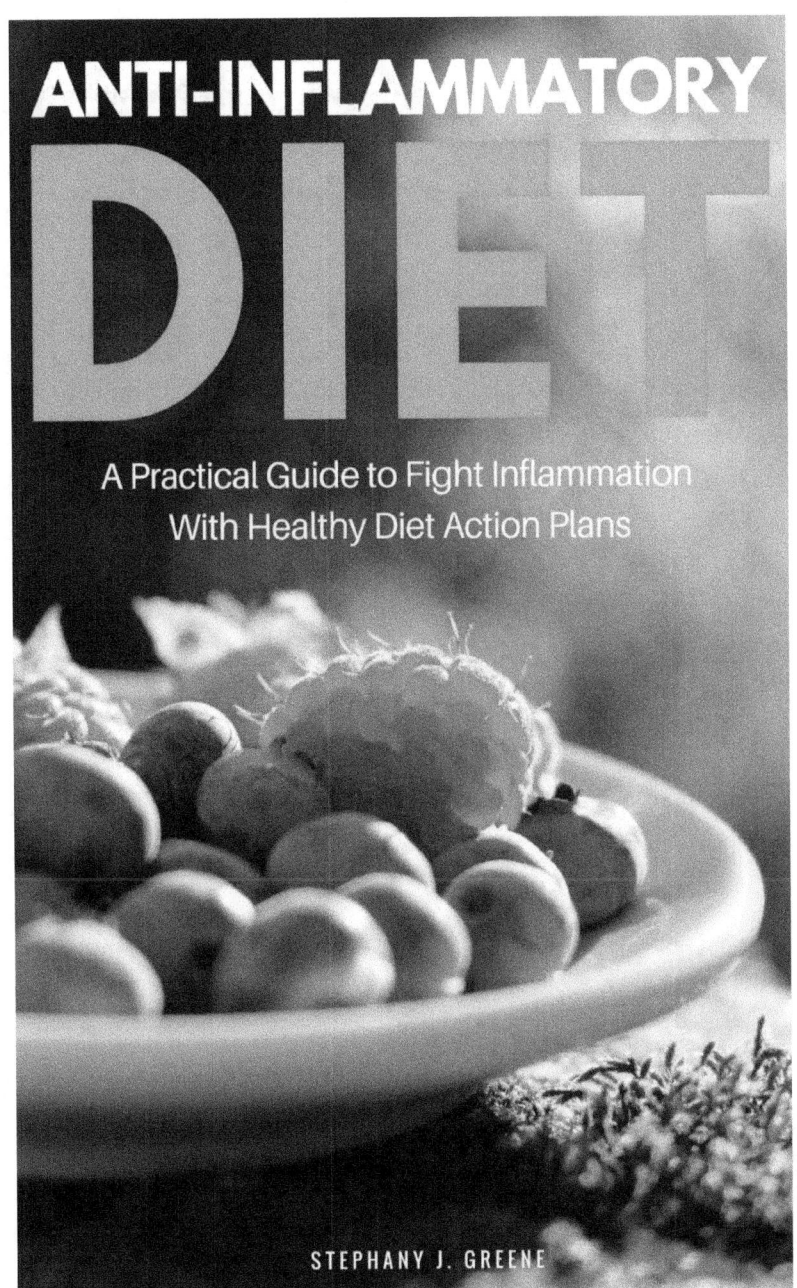

ANTI-INFLAMMATORY DIET

A Practical Guide to Fight Inflammation
With Healthy Diet Action Plans

STEPHANY J. GREENE

The book contains not only meal plans and ways to reduce inflammation in the body, but also some personal success stories that will help motivate you to change your dieting lifestyle. Next to this already available book, I also have a lot of other exciting book projects coming up soon. Improving your eating habits is always one of the most interesting things to write and read about, as it directly impacts our lives and health. So these next projects will certainly go more into moving towards a healthy lifestyle. Hope to see you around in another book of dieting wisdom!

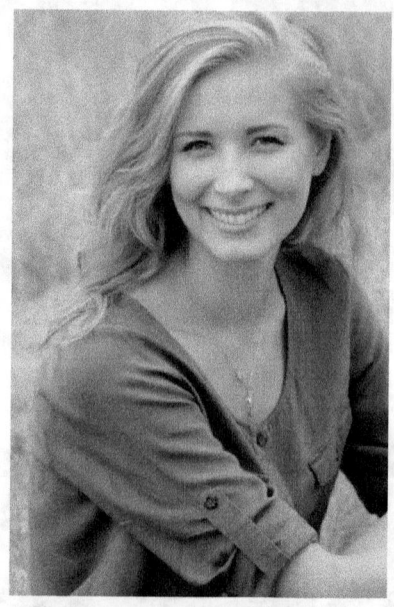

Stephany J. Greene

www.ingramcontent.com/pod-product-compliance
Lightning Source LLC
Chambersburg PA
CBHW062059280526
45788CB00003B/1287